To Celebrate

_____

_____

Date

_____

THANK YOU FOR COMING.

Let's celebrate!

Guest Name

_____

Wishes & Messages

_____

_____

_____

_____

_____

_____

_____

Email/Phone

Guest Name

Wishes & Messages

Email/Phone

Guest Name

Wishes & Messages

✉ Email/Phone

Guest Name

_____

Wishes & Messages

_____

_____

_____

_____

_____

_____

EMAIL/PHONE

Guest Name

_____

Wishes & Messages

_____

_____

_____

_____

_____

_____

_____

Email/Phone

Guest Name

_____

Wishes & Messages

_____

_____

_____

_____

_____

_____

Email/Phone

Guest Name

Wishes & Messages

_____

_____

_____

_____

_____

_____

_____

Email/Phone

Guest Name

Wishes & Messages

✉ EMAIL/PHONE

Guest Name

_____

Wishes & Messages

_____

_____

_____

_____

_____

_____

_____

Email/Phone

Guest Name

_____

Wishes & Messages

_____

_____

_____

_____

_____

_____

Email/Phone

Guest Name

_____

Wishes & Messages

_____

_____

_____

_____

_____

_____

_____

Email/Phone

Guest Name

_____

Wishes & Messages

_____

_____

_____

_____

_____

_____

Email/Phone

Guest Name

Wishes & Messages

Email/Phone

Guest Name

_____

Wishes & Messages

_____

_____

_____

_____

_____

_____

Email/Phone

Guest Name

Wishes & Messages

Email/Phone

Guest Name

_____

Wishes & Messages

_____

_____

_____

_____

_____

_____

Email/Phone

Guest Name

_____

Wishes & Messages

_____

_____

_____

_____

_____

_____

Email/Phone

Guest Name

_____

Wishes & Messages

_____

_____

_____

_____

_____

_____

Email/Phone

Guest Name

_____

Wishes & Messages

_____
_____
_____
_____
_____
_____
_____

Email/Phone

Guest Name

_____

Wishes & Messages

_____

_____

_____

_____

_____

_____

Email/Phone

Guest Name

_____

Wishes & Messages

_____

_____

_____

_____

_____

_____

Email/Phone

Guest Name

_____

Wishes & Messages

_____

_____

_____

_____

_____

_____

✉ Email/Phone

Guest Name

_____

Wishes & Messages

_____

_____

_____

_____

_____

_____

_____

Email/Phone

Guest Name

_____

Wishes & Messages

_____

_____

_____

_____

_____

_____

_____

Email/Phone

Guest Name

_____

Wishes & Messages

_____

_____

_____

_____

_____

_____

Email/Phone

Guest Name

Wishes & Messages

✉ E
Email/Phone

Guest Name

_____

Wishes & Messages

_____

_____

_____

_____

_____

_____

Email/Phone

Guest Name

Wishes & Messages

Email/Phone

Guest Name

_____

Wishes & Messages

_____

_____

_____

_____

_____

_____

Email/Phone

Guest Name

_____

Wishes & Messages

_____

_____

_____

_____

_____

_____

✉ Email/Phone

Guest Name

_____

Wishes & Messages

_____

_____

_____

_____

_____

_____

_____

Email/Phone

Guest Name

Wishes & Messages

Email/Phone

Guest Name

_____

Wishes & Messages

_____

_____

_____

_____

_____

_____

Email/Phone

Guest Name

_____

Wishes & Messages

_____

_____

_____

_____

_____

_____

Email/Phone

Guest Name

_____

Wishes & Messages

_____
_____
_____
_____
_____
_____
_____

Email/Phone

Guest Name

_____

Wishes & Messages

_____
_____
_____
_____
_____
_____

✉ Email/Phone

Guest Name

_____

Wishes & Messages

_____

_____

_____

_____

_____

_____

_____

Email/Phone

Guest Name

Wishes & Messages

Email/Phone

Guest Name

_____

Wishes & Messages

_____

_____

_____

_____

_____

_____

Email/Phone

Guest Name

Wishes & Messages

_____

_____

_____

_____

_____

_____

_____

EMAIL/PHONE

Guest Name

Wishes & Messages

Email/Phone

Guest Name

_____

Wishes & Messages

_____

_____

_____

_____

_____

_____

_____

Email/Phone

Guest Name

_____

Wishes & Messages

_____

_____

_____

_____

_____

_____

_____

Email/Phone

Guest Name

Wishes & Messages

_____

_____

_____

_____

_____

_____

Email/Phone

Guest Name

Wishes & Messages

Email/Phone

Guest Name

Wishes & Messages

Email/Phone

Guest Name

Wishes & Messages

Email/Phone

Guest Name

Wishes & Messages

_____

_____

_____

_____

_____

_____

_____

Email/Phone

Guest Name

_____

Wishes & Messages

_____

_____

_____

_____

_____

_____

Email/Phone

Guest Name

_____

Wishes & Messages

_____

_____

_____

_____

_____

_____

Email/Phone

Guest Name

_____

Wishes & Messages

_____

_____

_____

_____

_____

_____

_____

Email/Phone

Guest Name

Wishes & Messages

Email/Phone

Guest Name

_____

Wishes & Messages

_____

_____

_____

_____

_____

_____

Email/Phone

Guest Name

_____

Wishes & Messages

_____

_____

_____

_____

_____

_____

Email/Phone

Guest Name

_____

Wishes & Messages

_____

_____

_____

_____

_____

_____

_____

Email/Phone

Guest Name

Wishes & Messages

Email/Phone

Guest Name

_____

Wishes & Messages

_____

_____

_____

_____

_____

_____

Email/Phone

Guest Name

_____

Wishes & Messages

_____

_____

_____

_____

_____

_____

Email/Phone

Guest Name

Wishes & Messages

Email/Phone

Guest Name

_____

Wishes & Messages

_____
_____
_____
_____
_____
_____

Email/Phone

Guest Name

_____

Wishes & Messages

_____

_____

_____

_____

_____

_____

_____

Email/Phone

Guest Name

_____

Wishes & Messages

_____

_____

_____

_____

_____

_____

✉ Email/Phone

Guest Name

_____

Wishes & Messages

_____

_____

_____

_____

_____

_____

_____

✉ Email/Phone

Guest Name

_____

Wishes & Messages

_____

_____

_____

_____

_____

_____

Email/Phone

Guest Name

_____

Wishes & Messages

_____

_____

_____

_____

_____

_____

Email/Phone

Guest Name

_____

Wishes & Messages

_____

_____

_____

_____

_____

_____

Email/Phone

Guest Name

Wishes & Messages

Email/Phone

Guest Name

_____

Wishes & Messages

_____

_____

_____

_____

_____

_____

✉ Email/Phone

Guest Name

_____

Wishes & Messages

_____

_____

_____

_____

_____

_____

Email/Phone

Guest Name

_____

Wishes & Messages

_____

_____

_____

_____

_____

_____

Email/Phone

Guest Name

Wishes & Messages

_____

_____

_____

_____

_____

_____

_____

Email/Phone

Guest Name

_____

Wishes & Messages

_____

_____

_____

_____

_____

_____

Email/Phone

Guest Name

_____

Wishes & Messages

_____

_____

_____

_____

_____

_____

_____

Email/Phone

Guest Name

Wishes & Messages

_____

_____

_____

_____

_____

_____

_____

Email/Phone

Guest Name

_____

Wishes & Messages

_____
_____
_____
_____
_____
_____
_____

✉ Email/Phone

Guest Name

_____

Wishes & Messages

_____

_____

_____

_____

_____

_____

Email/Phone

Guest Name

_____

Wishes & Messages

_____

_____

_____

_____

_____

_____

Email/Phone

Guest Name

_____

Wishes & Messages

_____

_____

_____

_____

_____

_____

_____

Email/Phone

Guest Name

_____

Wishes & Messages

_____

_____

_____

_____

_____

_____

Email/Phone

Guest Name

Wishes & Messages

_____

_____

_____

_____

_____

_____

Email/Phone

Guest Name

_____

Wishes & Messages

_____

_____

_____

_____

_____

_____

Email/Phone

Guest Name

Wishes & Messages

Email/Phone

Guest Name

Wishes & Messages

Email/Phone

Guest Name

Wishes & Messages

Email/Phone

Guest Name

_____

Wishes & Messages

_____

_____

_____

_____

_____

_____

_____

Email/Phone

Guest Name

_____

Wishes & Messages

_____

_____

_____

_____

_____

_____

Email/Phone

Guest Name

_____

Wishes & Messages

_____

_____

_____

_____

_____

_____

_____

Email/Phone

Guest Name

_____

Wishes & Messages

_____

_____

_____

_____

_____

_____

Email/Phone

Guest Name

_____

Wishes & Messages

_____

_____

_____

_____

_____

_____

Email/Phone

Guest Name

Wishes & Messages

Email/Phone

Guest Name

_____

Wishes & Messages

_____

_____

_____

_____

_____

_____

_____

✉ Email/Phone

Guest Name

Wishes & Messages

Email/Phone

Guest Name

Wishes & Messages

Email/Phone

Guest Name

Wishes & Messages

Email/Phone

Guest Name

_____

Wishes & Messages

_____
_____
_____
_____
_____
_____
_____

✉ Email/Phone

Guest Name

Wishes & Messages

Email/Phone

Guest Name

_____

Wishes & Messages

_____

_____

_____

_____

_____

_____

Email/Phone

Guest Name

Wishes & Messages

Email/Phone

Guest Name

Wishes & Messages

✉️ Email/Phone

Guest Name

_____

Wishes & Messages

_____

_____

_____

_____

_____

_____

Email/Phone

Guest Name

Wishes & Messages

Email/Phone

Guest Name

Wishes & Messages

Email/Phone

Guest Name

_____

Wishes & Messages

_____

_____

_____

_____

_____

_____

_____

Email/Phone

Guest Name

Wishes & Messages

Email/Phone

Guest Name

_____

Wishes & Messages

_____

_____

_____

_____

_____

_____

_____

Email/Phone

NOTES & PHOTOS

NOTES & PHOTOS

NOTES & PHOTOS

NOTES & PHOTOS

NOTES & PHOTOS

GIFT LOG

Name / Email / Phone	Gift

GIFT LOG

Name / Email / Phone	Gift

GIFT LOG

Name /Email /Phone   **Gift**

GIFT LOG

Name / Email / Phone	Gift

GIFT LOG

Name / Email / Phone	Gift

GIFT LOG

Name / Email / Phone   *Gift*

Name / Email / Phone	Gift

GIFT LOG

Name / Email / Phone	Gift

CPSIA information can be obtained
at www.ICGtesting.com
Printed in the USA
LVHW061056150222
711186LV00010B/499